MIRACULOUS MICROBES

Billions and billions of healthy bacteria normally inhabit the human body and play a vital role in keeping us healthy. Among the most important is the bacteria *Lactobacillus acidophilus*, which is found most readily in some yogurts and in supplements. Essential for good digestion, acidophilus helps cure diarrhea and candida infections, lower cholesterol, prevent and heal cancer and restore healthy intestinal flora after antibiotic treatment.

ABOUT THE AUTHOR

Frank Murray is editorial director of *Let's Live* and *Nutrition Insights* magazines and editor-in-chief of *GreatLife* magazine and *Let's Live*/UK edition. In addition to writing the Keats Good Health Guide *Ginkgo Biloba* and being co-author of *Turmeric and the Healing Curcuminoids*, he has written several Keats books, including *The Big Family Guide to All the Minerals*.

Acidophilus and Your Health

The beneficial microorganisms that aid digestion and fight disease

Frank Murray

Keats Publishing, Inc. New Canaan, Connecticut

Acidophilus is intended solely for informational and educational purposes, and not as medical advice. Please consult a health professional if you have questions about your health.

7

Contents

Page

Introduction 6
The Benefits of Yogurt 9
  How to Make Yogurt 9
  How Accurate Are Yogurt Labels? 14
  Beneficial for All Ages 14
  Topical Uses of Yogurt 15
Two Men Behind the Microbes 17
Improving Digestion 18
  Billions and Billions of Bacteria 20
  Effects of Live Bacteria Products 25
  Colitis Treatment 26
Cancer and the Effects of Acidophilus 28
  Colon Cancer 30
  Breast Cancer 31
The Great Cholesterol Debate 32
Candida Albicans and Thrush 34
  How Acidophilus Can Help 35
  Dealing with Chronic Yeast Infections 37
Diarrhea 38
Replacing Intestinal Flora After Antibiotic Treatment 39
Other Conditions Helped by Acidophilus 41
References 43

For thousands of years microorganisms have contributed to humanity's existence through the preservation and processing of foods, the fixation of oxygen in the atmosphere so that plants can grow, the disposal of organic waste products and the manufacture of antibiotics. When microorganisms bioconvert foods into fermented or cultured products—yogurt, cheese, buttermilk, sauerkraut, pickles, cured meats and so on—lactic acid is produced by most of these cultures.

According to Marvin L. Speck, Ph.D. of North Carolina State University in Raleigh: "Certain lactic acid bacteria have established a beneficial ecological relationship with humans, which begins at the time of birth and persists throughout life. Especially important among these microorganisms are the lactobacilli. Soon after birth the digestive tract is colonized by a variety of microorganisms. Among the first are the lactobacilli which originate in the maternal vagina during the birth of the child. During [the mother's] puberty Doderlein's bacillus, which is considered to be identical with *Lactobacillus acidophilus*, establishes itself as a predominant vaginal microorganism. In addition to its microbial interactions, it provides inoculum to the infant during birth."[1]

As the infant breastfeeds, a stable microflora sets up housekeeping in the intestinal tract within a few days. Tests on the newborn's fecal contents have shown that the microflora are mostly *Lactobacillus bifidus* (bifidobacteria). For bottle-fed infants, the fecal microflora is similar to that of an adult.

While the stomach contains only a few indigenous organisms, the small intestine is the home of numerous bacterial flora, with *Lactobacillus acidophilus* being the most prominent.

This bacteria survives the passage through the powerful gastric juices in the stomach, and moves on to remain and grow in the intestines.

Our gastrointestinal tract normally contains more than 100 different strains of microorganisms, many of them numbering in the millions and billions. When you have a healthy contingent of intestinal flora, with the beneficial ones outnumbering the harmful ones, you can often escape some of the quite serious health problems that result when the situation is reversed.

In women, the normal vaginal flora includes *Lactobacillus acidophilus, Lactobacillus bifidus, Lactobacillus fermenti* and *Lactobacillus plantarum*. Abnormal flora sometimes found in the vagina include: *Candida albicans, Trichomonas vaginalis* and *Hemophilus vaginalis*. Because of antibiotics, hormonal imbalances, inadequate enemas, contacts with contaminated individuals and a defective immune system, these abnormal flora continue to grow, ostensibly because they have replaced the beneficial flora which have been killed off. Vaginitis can be treated with the appropriate lactobacilli and streptococci, because they inhibit the existing infection, restore the normal lactic acid flora and lower the pH of vaginal secretions to a normal level.[2]

As explained in this book, *Lactobacillus acidophilus* is one of the beneficial bacteria that are useful in fighting *Candida albicans* and thrush, two debilitating yeast infections that affect many women. These two infections are also a problem for patients of both sexes with acquired immune deficiency syndrome (AIDS); most holistic physicians prescribe *Lactobacillus acidophilus* to counteract these infections.

There are dozens of beneficial and harmful microorganisms which normally inhabit the gastrointestinal tract. According to Tomotori Mitsuoka, M.D. some of these are latent pathogenic bacteria, which invade the organs outside the intestinal tract and cause pathological symptoms when the individual's resistance is low. In fact, most of the bacteria separated from the focal infection (that is, localized) of sepsis, endocarditis, brain tumor, liver tumor, lung tumor, meningitis, urinary tract infection, cystitis, vaginitis, etc., are all resident intestinal bacteria. It is believed, Dr. Mitsuoka said, that some intestinal bacteria penetrate the intestinal walls and form focal places because of the administration of certain medicines, including antibiotics, cortisone and immunity-suppressing substances; radiation treatment; and physical and psychological stresses.[3]

Specific and nonspecific irritations of the defense system are not always a plus. For example, if some of the intestinal bacteria are associated with other antigens (that is, a substance that triggers the body to produce antibodies, as in an allergic reaction), they function as a common antigen against the infection and can result in asthma, rheumatism, etc.

Also, although a variety of live bacteria products are recommended for conditions such as diarrhea, constipation, dermatitis, gynecological problems, etc., an analysis of many of these products found that many were not of sufficient bacterial strength to be effective, according to G. Reuter. If such products are unable to pass through the stomach and duodenum and implant in the intestines, they are of little benefit, Reuter reported.

In the following chapters, you will be introduced to some of the beneficial lactic acid bacteria, such as *Lactobacillus acidophilus*, *Bifidobacterium bifidum* and *Streptococcus faecalis*, which are available commercially to control various diseases. As reported, researchers around the world are finding these beneficial bacteria to be highly effective in many cases of diarrhea, constipation, sluggish digestion, herpes simplex, some forms of cancer, in lowering cholesterol, for controlling yeast and so forth. For those taking antibiotics and other drugs, lactic acid bacteria are essential to restore these helpful microorganisms to the gastrointestinal tract and vagina after they have been inactivated by drugs. For those allergic to milk, milk-free acidophilus products are available. And for those with lactose intolerance, the lactic acid bacteria capsules can help correct this problem.

Gaylord Hauser did more than anyone to popularize the importance of yogurt in keeping the body healthy. In fact, his five "wonder foods," rich in the B vitamins, are ideal starting points for any healthful regimen. They are yogurt, brewer's yeast, powdered skim milk, wheat germ and blackstrap molasses.

'"You are as young as your colon, other scientists have said, notably the bacteriologist Metchnikoff," Hauser wrote in *Look Younger, Live Longer*. "He believed that the body is prematurely aged by toxic bacilli released by the decomposition of food in the bowels. His secret of youthfulness was to wage war on toxic bacilli in the colon by marshaling against them armies of the beneficent bacilli contained in acidophilus milk and yogurt."[1]

As reported elsewhere in this guide, not all commercial yogurts contain the helpful *Lactobacillus acidophilus* (it must be added at the proper time during processing), but yogurt does contain the beneficial *L. bulgaricus* and other bacilli, along with protein, calcium, vitamin B2 and other nutrients.

HOW TO MAKE YOGURT

Hauser's favorite way of making yogurt at home was to beat into one pint of water these ingredients:

1½ cups powdered skim milk
3 tbsp previously made yogurt or commercial yogurt (as a starter)
1 large can evaporated milk

When this mixture is beaten smooth, add 1 quart of water and pour into serving glasses. Set these glasses in a large pan with enough warm water to reach the top of the glasses. Place the pan over a warming unit, pilot light or simmer burner to maintain the temperature of the water between 105 and 124° F. (Or use a yogurt maker.) The yogurt should thicken and be ready to chill in about three hours. If it takes longer, the temperature was probably not maintained correctly. After chilling, serve plain, with chives or other herbs, with fresh or canned fruit, or sweetened with maple syrup, honey or blackstrap molasses.

"Yogurt is a 'must' on the Live Longer diet," Hauser continued. "Among the Bulgarians, where yogurt is a part of each meal but where diet is not outstanding in other aspects, the life span is longer than that of any other people in the world; Bulgarians are credited with retaining vigor and virility and the characteristics of youth to an extremely advanced age."

Yogurt is also an excellent food for those who are ill, since the milk proteins are already partially digested by bacterial enzymes during the culturing process and the milk calcium has been dissolved in the lactic acid of the yogurt, making it easier to absorb. In the intestinal tract, the bacteria help check the growth of putrefactive and pathological organisms which cause discomfort and gas.

This "wonder food" has been around at least 4,000 years. Legend has it that Abraham was taught to make this fermented milk product by an angel. According to another tale, yogurt was discovered in the Middle East by a hungry nomad who had packed some milk away in a goatskin bag while traveling by camel across the desert. When he later opened the bag, he found a thick, tart custard, which was formed by bacteria thriving on milk sugar in the heat of the sun.[2]

Meg Cadou Hirshberg, author of *The Stonyfield Farm Yogurt Cookbook*, wrote: "In many societies yogurt is more than just another food. This cultured product is . . . an important part of many cultures, with recipes and bacterial 'starters' handed down through the generations. In many societies, yogurt and other cultured milk products (such as kefir) have been long thought to have therapeutic and life-enhancing properties."

Hirshberg offers this advice for buying yogurt:

1. Always look for yogurt with "live, active cultures" noted on the label. Some manufacturers pasteurize their yogurts after the beneficial bacteria have been added, thereby prolonging the product's shelf life but killing the bacteria that provide many of yogurt's health benefits.

2. Look for yogurt to which the beneficial *Lactobacillus acidophilus* bacterium has been added. Most yogurts do not contain *Lactobacillus acidophilus*, but it forms more than half of the bacterial culture in one brand.

3. Avoid Swiss or pudding-style yogurts. These are fermented in vats and then transferred to the cups in which they are sold. This process breaks the gel, so that artificial binders and stabilizers must be added.

Buy yogurt made from unhomogenized milk. Homogenization is practiced by most yogurt manufacturers and is often confused with pasteurization, though the two actually have nothing in common. Homogenization involves forcing milk through tiny openings that break up the milk fat or cream so that it becomes evenly mixed throughout the product. In unhomogenized yogurt, the cream simply rises to the top, just as it used to in old-fashioned milk bottles, and the cultures are subject to less time and handling during processing.

Read the label to see what sweeteners have been used. Many consumers prefer to avoid sugar or artificial sweeteners and look for yogurt with honey or natural fruit juice as a sweetener.

Yogurt labels may not tell the complete story. As explained by one major manufacturer, today's production facilities are a mixture of clinical laboratories, sophisticated dairy machinery, along with temperature-controlled refrigerators and incubators. New technologies are combined with personal care, and the various steps necessary for producing yogurt are conducted in a scientifically purified atmosphere. Some manufacturers fill yogurt containers cup by cup; others do it in large batches. Some brands of yogurt contain artificial preservatives to prolong shelf life. Some yogurts are made from partially skimmed milk, others from whole milk.

Juan E. Metzger, board chairman of one yogurt manufacturing company, said, "Yogurt helps people to lose weight and also helps in a weight-maintenance program. An 8-oz. serving of our plain variety yields 150 calories, 12 grams of protein for body building and maintenance, 17 grams of carbohydrates for energy and 4 grams of fat. It also provides 30 percent of the riboflavin (B2), and 40 percent of the calcium, 35 percent of the phosphorus and 20 percent of vitamin B12, according to U.S. Recommended Daily Allowances."[3]

Yogurt may enhance immunity, according to Sheldon Saul Hendler, M.D., Ph.D. in *The Purification Prescription*. A U.S. Department of Agriculture study compared two groups of rats injected with large doses of Salmonella. One group had been fed yogurt prior to injection; the other group, milk. The rats fed yogurt did not get nearly as sick as those fed milk and fewer of them died. In a Romanian study, Dr. Hendler reported, yogurt appeared to protect mice against influenza. Yogurt has been used to treat diarrhea that is secondary to bacterial infection or that is associated with antibiotic use, ulcerative colitis and diverticulitis. Also, yogurt does contain some substances that have antibiotic activity. Recently, Italian scientists have shown that yogurt has immune-enhancing effects in experimental animals and humans. There is even evidence that yogurt and acidophilus milk are protective against colon cancer.[4]

"Fermented milk products, such as yogurt, taken daily can help restore a normal intestinal flora and possibly help in the healing process of the 'leaky-gut' syndrome common in alcoholism," Dr. Hendler continued. "Fermented milk products contain lactic acid, which causes their sour taste. Lactic acid has healing properties for dry skin and may have similar healing power in the intestine."

In *Yogurt: Nutritional and Health Properties*, Robert L. Sellars stated that, for maximum benefit, yogurt should not be heated before being consumed. Heating inactivates the beneficial bacteria that contribute to good health. Unheated yogurt provides these healthful properties:

1. Promotes growth.
2. Aids in lactose digestion.
3. Increases mineral absorption.
4. Contains antimicrobial factors.
5. Contains anticarcinogenic factors.
6. Stimulates immunological response system.
7. Stimulates reduction of blood serum cholesterol.[5]

Several researchers have reported on the reduced level of lactose in yogurt during manufacture, Sellars said. This reduction is associated with an increase in the residual level of lactase, the enzyme produced by the starter cultures necessary for making yogurt. Lactase is responsible for the conversion of lactose or milk sugar to lactic acid, which lowers the pH and causes the milk casein to coagulate.

When yogurt is not heated, lactase is present in the yogurt when it's eaten, and since it survives in the intestinal tract, it offers those who are lactose intolerant an opportunity to consume fermented yogurt without experiencing the discomfort that they have when eating dairy products.

"The production of lactic acid during the manufacture of yogurt is important not only to meet commercial requirements during manufacture, but to provide the following," Sellars added: "1) acts as a preservative; 2) contributes a mildly sour but refreshing taste; 3) enhances digestibility of casein (milk protein); 4) improves utilization and absorption of minerals; 5) increases metabolism of oné or two isometric forms of lactic acid; and 6) enhances relaxation and peristalsis. Without the above attributes yogurt would not be safe, or have the shelf stability demanded by consumers. Nor would it have a pleasant and refreshing taste. Also, it would not be as easily digestible, display improved absorption of minerals and enhanced relaxation for improved peristalsis (natural movement of digestive substances through the gut) once in the intestines."

Dairy foods, and particularly fermented ones like yogurt, acidophilus/yogurt, cultured buttermilk and cheese, serve as excellent dietary sources of calcium, not only because of their high calcium content but also because of its excellent bioavailability in these foods. Sellars said that since the calcium ion becomes more solubilized at acid pH's, cultured-fermented dairy foods are excellent sources of dietary calcium and yogurt is one of the best sources.

In the processing of fruit-flavored yogurts, the highly processed fruit (usually a jam or jelly) is placed in yogurt tubs but kept physically separate from the bacteria in the milk, which is incubating and fermenting. A barrier of chemicals is placed above the fruit layer to buffer it. If this were not done, the bacteria in the culture would begin digesting the fruit and its sugar and would thus inhibit the fermenting of the milk. Leon Chaitow, M.D., D.O. and Natasha Trenev suggest in *ProBiotics* that consumers buy yogurts with live cultures and add their own fresh fruit as they eat it instead.[6]

HOW ACCURATE ARE YOGURT LABELS?

An analysis of 12 yogurt products from a variety of commercial outlets showed that all the labels stated that the yogurt contained *Lactobacillus acidophilus,* according to *ProBiotics.* Then two researchers investigated.

The first stage of the test was to see whether whatever organisms (if any) were in the products could survive the digestive acids they would meet after being eaten. Out of 12 products only five contained bile-resistant organisms, and only three of these actually contained any *Lactobacillus acidophilus.* So, less than half of the products assessed in this admittedly small survey had any live cultures which might survive the stomach and small intestine, and a mere quarter contained what the label stated was the active culture in the product.

What about frozen yogurt? The nutritive value of this snack is tarnished by the addition of vast quantities of either sugar or artificial sweeteners, also coloring, flavoring and stabilizing chemicals. Plus the quality of milk used may be poor. It's better to make your own iced yogurt at home.

BENEFICIAL FOR ALL AGES

Many adults lose their taste or tolerance for milk with age, but yogurt continues to agree with them on both counts.

That makes yogurt an ideal calcium source for the over-21 set, as well as children.[7]

Even lactose-intolerant people absorbed the calcium from yogurt as well as the calcium from milk, according to a study done at the Veterans Administration Medical Center in Minneapolis. Also in a study of 3,000 government workers done by Erasmus University in the Netherlands, those who ate yogurt, along with whole-grain bread, porridge, vegetables, fruit and fish had better survival rates than subjects who did not follow this regimen.

TOPICAL USES OF YOGURT

Writing in *Essential Supplements for Women*, Carolyn Reuben, C.A. and Joan Priestly, M.D. reported that a vaginal douche using unflavored yogurt (preferably made at home) is often useful in treating stubborn cases of vaginitis.[8] As reported previously, the vagina normally contains large amounts of *Lactobacillus acidophilus* and other beneficial organisms, and when they are in short supply, serious consequences can result.

Acidophilus is the organism that usually keeps the infectious agents in the vagina in line. However, when you take antibiotics, or when the vaginal pH changes for whatever reason, the "good guys" are killed off or their numbers are diminished and the "baddies" overwhelm the area. By reintroducing cultures of *Lactobacillus acidophilus*, you can rebalance the microorganism menagerie and restore peace within, the authors said.

If you use commercially prepared yogurt, recommended brands include Continental and Alta-Dena that contain live *Lactobacillus acidophilus* cultures. For vaginal application you can purchase *Lactobacillus acidophilus* culture in liquid form at a health food store. Be sure to keep it refrigerated.

A combination of yogurt and cranberry juice is often useful in treating urinary tract infections common to women, the authors added. The yogurt is either eaten or applied to the vulval area. The cranberry juice, rich in vitamin C, is drunk.

Since yogurt, either consumed or applied topically, is a valuable substance for providing many health benefits, we should include it in our meals regularly. Although it adds a tangy taste to cooked recipes, it should be mentioned that many of the beneficial bacteria are probably destroyed by the heat. But you can still benefit from other substances that are found in yogurt. Here are some tasty recipes.

Breakfast Boost
2 containers (8 oz. each) unflavored (plain) yogurt
hulled strawberries and/or sliced, peeled bananas
⅓ cup cold milk
3 tbsp honey
2 tbsp orange juice
2 ice cubes
Place ingredients in blender and cover. Blend until smooth and frothy. Serve in chilled glasses. Serves three.

Fruity Frapp
1 container (8 oz.) unflavored yogurt
boysenberries
¾ cup cold milk
½ cup fresh strawberries, hulled
Place ingredients in a blender and cover. Blend until smooth and frothy. Serve in chilled glasses. Serves two.

For those who have not acquired a taste for yogurt, why not give this healthful food another try? It is versatile and nutritious, providing a wealth of nutrients that we need each day. The most delicious yogurt I have ever tasted was in Bulgaria—where else?—where it was made with water buffalo milk. The rich, creamy yogurt was definitely ambrosia for the gods.

TWO MEN BEHIND THE MICROBES

Although Elie Metchnikoff, M.D. is often regarded as the Father of Acidophilus, his studies involving yogurt and fermented milk were generally concerned with *Lactobacillus bulgaricus* and other strains of the Lactobacillus family, rather than *Lactobacillus acidophilus*, which is not a normal constituent in yogurt but is sometimes added to commercial products.

Born May 15, 1845, in Ivanovka, Kharkov, Russia, Metchnikoff, after finishing his studies, was invited to Paris to work with Louis Pasteur in 1888. Metchnikoff succeeded Pasteur as head of the Pasteur Institute in 1895 and remained its director until his death in 1916.

Metchnikoff's studies were far-ranging and included zoology, pathology, the anatomy of vertebrates, embryology and longevity especially as it relates to healthy bacteria in the alimentary canal. In 1908, he and Paul Ehrlich received the Nobel Prize for medicine. Among Metchnikoff's many findings was the first proof that lactobacilli could transform lactose in milk into lactic acid and that lactic acid suppressed or killed disease-causing organisms in milk or milk products treated with lactobacilli.[1] Doctors began to recommend sour milk to patients as a hygienic food, and easy-to-use preparations of "friendly bacteria" have since been widely used to prevent and cure a variety of health problems.

Leo F. Rettger, M.D. did definitive work on *Lactobacillus acidophilus* in landmark studies as a professor of bacteriology at Yale University in New Haven, Connecticut. His interest in intestinal flora began about 1912 when he found a correlation between lactose and dextrin feeding and an increase in *Lactobacillus acidophilus* in the intestines. Rettger's studies indicated that acidophilus was superior to bulgaricus as a "persisting organism in the intestine," and it was acidophilus that he used for his thesis that these organisms could prevent the growth of disease-causing bacteria.

Rettger and colleagues found that milk cultures of acidophilus were especially effective in transforming human intestinal flora. Furthermore, this lactic acid bacteria was more easily cultivated than others, and once implanted in the gut, it remains there and grows. This research explains why so many modern-day physicians recommend *Lactobacillus acidophilus* as a means of promoting normal digestion and why this friendly bacteria can prevent or treat a variety of ills.

IMPROVING DIGESTION

Measuring from 25 to 30 feet in length, the digestive system is literally a long tube stretching from the mouth to the anus. After food and beverages are ingested, they travel through the mouth, esophagus, stomach, small intestine, large intestine, the rectum and then are discharged as fecal matter by the anus. As it travels this route, food is broken down for easier digestion by salivary glands, the gall bladder, liver and the pancreas.[1]

The style of eating has a major effect on one component of the gastrointestinal tract, the bacterial flora, according to Abram Hoffer, M.D., Ph.D. in *Orthomolecular Medicine for Physicians*. Living food has a low bacteria count, since there has been little time for bacteria to grow, and the number of bacteria is further diminished by the hydrochloric acid in the stomach.[2]

"Acid-tolerant bacteria, such as acidophilus, are able to survive passage through the stomach," wrote Hoffer. "Once the food has passed into the small intestine, its pH becomes alkaline. The warm body temperature, moisture and ample food provide an ideal medium for bacteria; they thrive. The further down the GI tract, the more bacteria are present. The upper intestine should have fewer bacteria than 10,000 per ml. The bulk of the weight of the feces is bacteria."

The bacteria count is reduced, at least in the upper part of the GI tract, by strong stomach acids. Therefore, those who lack sufficient amounts of acid are more apt to suffer bacterial overgrowth, with yeast cells among them. The ileocecal valve prevents the reflux of material into the upper intestine, while bacteria are also suppressed by the secretion of bile and pancreatic juices into the duodenum. Since these juices are sterile, they aid in digesting bacterial cells. Finally, steady peristalsis propels the GI contents onward, further diminishing bacterial growth. The growth of bacteria is highest in the colon and rectum, and lowest in the duodenum.

Harmful bacteria not only interfere with the absorption of nutrients, they produce toxins that injure intestinal walls, interfering with the absorption of nutrients and water.

Dr. Hoffer added: "The body adapted to the inevitable bacterial growth by allowing its maximum growth in an area where there is the least absorption, that is, in the colon. By the time food reaches the colon most of the soluble nutrients have been extracted. Once in the colon, where bacterial growth is at its greatest, much less harm comes to the body. A high-fiber diet stimulates peristalsis, moving the food through within a day or so. The colon is evacuated normally about twice a day. Constipated people may require three days or more, and some have one bowel movement once every seven days, providing much more time for bacterial growth."

The longer that fecal matter remains in the digestive system, the greater the chances for harmful carcinogens to build up. When digestion purrs along at a normal rate, often helped by friendly bacteria such as *Lactobacillus acidophilus*, harmful bacteria are less likely to cause damage to the digestive tract. As Hoffer suggested, bowel movements are an individual matter, and what may be considered constipation by one person may be simply a normal routine for someone else. The size and appearance of the stool are generally the bottom line (no pun intended). A pencil-thin stool or small, pebbly discharges are cause for concern. One of the most counterproductive measures you can take is regular laxative use, since they interfere with the normal routine of digestion, may be habit forming and dispatch much-needed vitamins, minerals, beneficial bacteria and other necessary constituents.

In addition to constipation, a malfunctioning digestive tract can produce a variety of painful and unpleasant disorders, most of which are related to diet and lifestyle. These include anal abscesses and fistulas, appendicitis, Crohn's disease, diverticulitis, gallbladder disease, gastritis, gastroenteritis, hemorrhoids, hiatal hernia, irritable bowel syndrome, pancreatitis, ulcerative colitis, varicose veins and other conditions. The malabsorption of food or allergic reactions to certain foods can result in celiac disease, lactose intolerance, gluten intolerance and others. Digestion may also be impaired by tumors, radiotherapy and numerous other things.

"In the Western world the average weight of the daily stool is about 3 ounces (100 grams), though weight increases if the diet has more vegetables, fruit and bran," said Christiaan Barnard, M.D. in *The Body Machine*. "The rural African or Asian, on a high natural fiber diet, may pass up to 16 ounces (500 grams) of feces a day. It takes between 12 and 24 hours for matter to pass from one end of the large intestine to the other. In contrast, it takes between 2 and 6 hours for matter to pass through the stomach and a further 5 to 6 hours for it to pass through the small intestine."[3]

Because of the germ-free environment of the uterus, babies are born without any microorganisms in their alimentary canal. As babies begin to eat, however, microorganisms take up residence in the stomach and intestines. At first there is a difference between breast-fed and bottle-fed babies, with the former having a higher proportion of lactobacilli and lactic acid streptococci, and the bottle-fed infants a more varied range of bacteria.[4]

BILLIONS AND BILLIONS OF BACTERIA

The amount of bacteria present in the digestive system is so huge, they are counted in powers of 10; 10^3 is 1,000 and 10^6 is 1,000,000. In the esophagus, the numbers are 10^3 to 10^6

per gram of contents. In the small intestine there are about 10^5 to 10^8 bacteria per gram, and this increases in the large intestine or colon to 10^8 to 10^{11}. In the feces, 10 or 20 percent of the weight consists of bacteria, most of which are anaerobic; that is, they can grow without oxygen.

The huge numbers of bacteria in the colon actively affect the other constituents of the gut. These are mostly harmless bacteria which tend to reduce the number of pathogenic organisms entering the gut. Without these beneficial bacteria, we would be much more susceptible to intestinal infection. The helpful bacteria also synthesize vitamin K and some of the B vitamins, thus making us less dependent on dietary sources of these vitamins. The use of antibiotics and other drugs inhibits the amount of vitamins supplied by the bacteria, increasing our need for these nutrients. Bacteria also digest small amounts of some of the constituents of dietary fiber, enabling them to be absorbed. Still another function of intestinal bacteria is to break down bile pigments and bile acids.

You can change the relative proportions of bacteria in the colon by including fairly large amounts of yogurt in your diet. But since bacteria revert to original distribution when you stop eating yogurt, the change is temporary.

Unless there is a steady supply of *Lactobacillus acidophilus* and other beneficial bacteria in the gut, we cannot properly benefit from these intestinal flora. For those who do not wish to eat yogurt on a regular basis, because of the taste or the calories, supplements of acidophilus and other useful bacteria are a logical choice. Because of the countless numbers of bacteria in these supplements, they implant in the gut and vagina and keep the alimentary canal in a healthy state.

Research studies have shown these impressive results in treating digestive disorders with acidophilus supplements:

- The successful implantation of *Lactobacillus acidophilus* provided relief in mucous colitis, irritable colon, idiopathic ulcerative colitis and other problems associated with constipation, according to L. F. Rettger and colleagues in *Lactobacillus acidophilus: Its Therapeutic Application*.[5,6]
- In 356 cases of chronic constipation, 305 responded favorably to supplementation with acidophilus.[7] Articles in *Archives of Internal Medicine* also demonstrated the beneficial

effects of acidophilus, although results were sometimes not apparent for a few weeks or months.[8,9]

- Fifteen of 21 patients with constipation and diarrhea improved with acidophilus; 46 of 50 cases of functiona_ diarrhea responded to the supplement; and 32 of 39 patients with irritable colon and diverticulitis improved.[10]
- A study reported in *Clinical Pediatrics* found that 45 infants ranging in age from 1 to 27 months with infantile diarrhea improved with yogurt or Neomycin-kaopectate. However, those receiving the yogurt recovered more rapidly.[11]
- In a study using acidophilus tablets, excellent results were observed in most of the 56 patients with chronic constipation, functional diarrhea, mucous colitis and megacolon, according to Asher Winkelstein, M.D. in *American Practitioner and Digest of Treatment.*[12]
- According to the *American Journal of Gastroenterology*, 32 of 39 patients treated with acidophilus tablets for irritable colon (31) and diverticulitis (8) found improvement within one to three weeks of treatment. Their symptoms had included abdominal pain, constipation, diarrhea (or alternating constipation and diarrhea) and gas.
- "There was gratifying improvement" in 15 of 18 patients who were given acidophilus tablets to treat irritable bowel, diarrhea or constipation, diverticulitis and neurosis, Dr. Winkelstein reported. "These patients stated that they were pleased with their improved bowel regularity and clearing up of other complaints (for example, abdominal pain)."[12]

Normally, the principal inhabitants of the intestine are *E. coli*, the enterococcus and *Lactobacillus acidophilus*. The first two are putrefactive bacteria which break down protein in the intestine, thereby liberating toxins that are usually detoxified by the liver. Winkelstein believes these toxic amines form protein putrefaction; then *E. coli* and its soluble toxin may attach and harm the liver, perhaps resulting in subclinical hepatitis. These products are certainly implicated in damaging an already diseased liver, Winkelstein said. Since it is possible that this damage impairs the detoxifying function of the liver, it would seem prudent in all types of liver disease to supplant putrefactive organisms in the bowel with *Lactobacillus acidophilus.*

On the other hand, the physician noted, acidophilus is a fermentative organism which merely produces lactic acid. This supposedly weak acid inhibits the growth of *E. coli* and holds it in check so its putrefactive function is not carried too far, possibly damaging the liver or allowing absorption of toxic substances into the bloodstream. A high-protein diet is conducive to a preponderance of *E. coli* in the intestinal flora, while a high-carbohydrate diet favors the growth of fermentative organisms.

Winkelstein prescribed *Lactobacillus acidophilus* tablets for 107 patients. Good symptomatic responses were obtained in 45 of 49 cases of chronic constipation; 16 of 17 cases of functional diarrhea; four of five cases of mucous colitis; and all 13 cases of antibiotic colitis, as well as eight cases of sigmoid diverticulitis and four cases of megacolon, he said. As might be expected, he added, seven cases of ulcerative colitis and a few miscellaneous conditions (two rheumatoid arthritis, one ileitis and one vertigo) failed to respond.

George Von Hilsheimer, Ph.D. is quoted in *The Yeast Connection: A Medical Breakthrough* as saying: "Observations of a long series of psychiatric patients disclosed a deficiency of *Lactobacillus acidophilus* in their stools associated with GI symptoms and other evidences of idiosyncratic responses to food . . . . Supplementation with high levels of *Lactobacillus acidophilus* in the form of freeze-dried capsules, cultured milk, yogurt or 'sweet acidophilus' milk resulted in grossly observable changes in stool, increase in stool *Lactobacillus acidophilus*, and reductions of symptoms associated with food."[13]

Malodorous gases which are passed in the flatus are not swallowed air but are probably colon bacteria acting on fats, according to James L. A. Roth, M.D. reporting in *Medical World News* in 1975. He added that *Lactobacillus acidophilus* is beneficial because there is less fermentation and, therefore, less likelihood of flatulence.[14]

Although *L. acidophilus* and *Bifidobacterium bifidum* are normal inhabitants of the GI tract, several groups of people are often deficient or devoid of the two bacteria, such as formula-fed infants, the elderly and those suffering from intestinal ill-nesses. Their digestion can reportedly be improved by the intake of acidophilus, which is said to restore the GI tract's bacterial population, according to *Diveronmental Nutrition*.[15]

"Because breast-fed babies have such inoffensive-smelling stools, attempts have been made to imitate the bacteria in their intestines," reported Lendon Smith, M.D. in *Feed Your-self Right*. "Capsules with live *Lactobacillus acidophilus* can be swallowed in the hope that these good bacteria will set up housekeeping. They help produce an acid stool with a buffering ability (acetic acid and acetate), and with low counts of *E. coli* and putrefactive bacteria. Enthusiastic users of *Lactobacillus acidophilus* say that gas is less, canker sores disappear, and energy improves. It's cheap and safe, but may have to be reswallowed periodically. Those with diarrhea that is unresponsive to antibiotics often improve with *Lactobacillus acidophilus*."[16]

Henry D. Isenberg, Ph.D. of Long Island Jewish-Hillside Medical Center, New York, said that *Lactobacillus acidophilus* helps to maintain our ecological balance, and it achieves this end within the intimate human biosphere by curtailing putrefaction. "This process of incomplete anaerobic microbial decay is favored by our changing food customs, by the advances in food processing and by the addition of antimicrobial agents, all of which disrupt the quite delicate equilibrium so essential for the proper functioning of our body."[17]

Eugene R. Jolly, M.D., Ph.D., who had been introduced to *Lactobacillus acidophilus* many years ago, added that, at that time, it was clear that there was a notable therapeutic potential for such products as adjuncts in the treatment of a number of gastrointestinal disorders, such as irritable bowel syndrome, chronic constipation and chronic diarrhea, as well as other more severe forms of GI complaints.

"At the time, at the Food and Drug Administration, it seemed to us that a good *Lactobacillus acidophilus* product would certainly be a boon to our entire population, particularly people dependent on laxatives or those who complained constantly of just plain indigestion," Dr. Jolly said. He added that it was difficult to pinpoint when digestive benefits from lactobacilli were first noted, but the feeding of buttermilk to infants was a long-established custom in Holland. Around the turn of the century, this method of treating infantile diarrhea was imported to the U.S. and buttermilk became an important therapeutic aid in pediatric medicine.

Around 1914, it was proven that when *Lactobacillus acidophilus* was fed to humans it would implant in the intestines, improving bowel function and digestion in those with chronic digestive disorders. Researchers believed that acidophilus worked by suppressing the putrefactive, gas-forming and disease-promoting bacteria. It was important that acidophilus be used in relatively large amounts, and that only the live, active culture was effective.[17]

Much more recently, Max A. Tesler, M.D. said that past and present microbiological research indicates the effectiveness of acidophilus in a wide variety of functional and organic gastrointestinal conditions. In particular, irritable bowel syndrome characterized by an imbalance of bacterial flora.

"It is obvious that promoting normal bacterial function and diminishing the use of laxatives or other artificial bowel stimulants and allowing broader food tolerance for a large number of people is a most desirable endpoint," Dr. Tesler said. "It is thus far more desirable to treat a condition by restoring the intestine to its more natural state, rather than treat the symptoms of the condition artificially by laxatives or antidiarreal agents, which do not serve to correct the underlying problem and may become habit-forming and symptom-producing in their own right."

EFFECTS OF LIVE BACTERIA PRODUCTS

There are seven effects of live bacteria products such as acidophilus:
1. Intestine normalization and suppression of putrefaction
2. Suppression of the growth of pathogenic bacteria and putrefactive bacteria
3. Increased resistance against infections

4. Production of lactic acid, acetic acid, butyric acid and antibiotics
5. Synthesis of vitamins B1, B2, B6 and nicotinic acid amide
6. Formation of a medium that is favorable for the growth of bifidus bacteria
7. A variety of other miscellaneous applications

"Among the many kinds of lactic acid bacteria," Japanese researchers reported in New Medicines and Clinics, "it is considered that those residing in the human gastrointestinal tract are more effective than others. The effects of lactic acid on constipation include the production of lactic acid and acetic acid and the adherence to the intestinal tract mucus. Faecalis bacteria grow rapidly, make the content of the intestinal tract acidic and help useful bacteria grow, such as acidophilus and bifidus bacteria, which are relatively slow to grow. The capability of faecalis bacteria in adhering to the intestinal tract mucosa is higher than that of acidophilus bacteria."[18]

However, they added, among lactic acid bacteria, acidophilus bacteria have the best capability in producing lactic acid and thus have a better capability of maintaining the content of the intestinal tract's acetic acid than do faecalis bacteria.

COLITIS TREATMENT

Lactobacillus acidophilus supplements, in either capsule or liquid form, have given relief to many patients with colitis. In addition, the eating of several small, frequent meals during the course of the day is better than burdening the digestive system with three large meals. Colitis is an inflammation of the large bowel or colon, which can sometimes be very serious. It is also painful.

Although the cause of chronic colitis or ulcerative colitis is unknown, physicians must take care to distinguish true colitis from such common conditions as diverticular disease, irritable bowel and spastic colon. As an example, the pangs produced in those who are lactose intolerant can sometimes be misdiagnosed as colitis. The latter conditions are more a matter of function, and are more easily treated, whereas colitis involves serious physical damage to the colon.

One patient with colitis-like symptoms was hospitalized for several days and given a battery of tests. After being told he had ulcerative colitis, he was put on a soft, bland diet. When his symptoms of pain and diarrhea did not go away, he saw a gastroenterologist, who diagnosed lactose intolerance. When the patient stopped eating dairy products, his symptoms disappeared and his colon returned to normal.[19]

According to *The New England Journal of Medicine* (April 23, 1981), methyldopa, a drug used to treat high blood pressure, has been associated with acute cases of colitis. Numerous other studies have linked a type of colitis called pseudomembranous colitis to antibiotics such as clindamycin, lincomycin, tetracycline, ampicillin, penicillin and others. This form of colitis is potentially fatal in the elderly, the November 1979 *Geriatrics* reported.

Barbara Solomon, M.D. of Baltimore, Maryland, noted that, in susceptible people, allergic reactions to commonly eaten foods can cause ulcerative colitis and Crohn's disease, another inflammatory disease of the bowel. She believes that patients with ulcerative colitis are often allergic to dairy products, wheat, oats, barley, rye and/or corn. When these and any other suspect foods are eliminated, the patient often responds favorably.

"The colitis sufferer should be on a totally high-nutrition diet to give (the patient's) body every chance to heal itself." Reduced absorption of vitamin A has been reported in colitis and that vitamin is very important in maintaining strong epithelium (the intestinal lining). Zinc is also important in healing chronic ulcerations of epithelial tissue, and vitamin C is necessary to build new tissue, as are amino acids from protein. In addition, colitis patients need pantothenic acid, one of the B vitamins also known as the anti-stress vitamin.[19]

Folic acid is another vital B vitamin which is often found to be severely lacking in colitis patients. It can be replaced by increasing the intake of foods rich in this nutrient, or by using folic acid supplements. Complicating the cure or control of colitis is that sulfasalazine, the drug most widely used to treat colitis, is also responsible for interfering with the absorption of folate, according to *The New England Journal of Medicine*, Dec. 17, 1981.

While *Lactobacillus acidophilus* and other beneficial lactic acid bacteria help to normalize digestion, they are not the only players. Vitamins, minerals, amino acids and other nutrients also play a major role. In addition, the overuse of laxatives and drugs and some inherited conditions should also be considered as potential causes of tummy troubles.

CANCER AND THE EFFECTS OF ACIDOPHILUS

Second only to heart disease as a cause of death in the United States, cancer claims almost 500,000 lives annually. An estimated one in four people will eventually develop one of the over 100 forms of cancer, and approximately one out of every six deaths in the U.S. will be due to cancer.

Since the ancient Greeks determined that spreading cancerous tumors resembled the claws of a crab, they referred to the crablike disease as *karkinos*. This was translated into Latin as *cancer*. Cancer is a group of diseases involving an abnormal, unrestricted growth of body cells.[1]

The billions of cells inside our bodies grow rapidly during childhood, but, as we reach maturity, cells divide and reproduce only to replace worn-out cells or to repair wounds. However, cancer cells multiply rapidly and use nourishment that is needed by healthy cells. During its accelerated growth, the cancerous cells break away from the original cancer mass and by way of the bloodstream or lymphatic system move to other parts of the body. In their new locations the cancer cells form secondary sites or metastases and if significant organs such as the liver or kidneys are invaded, life expectancy is greatly diminished.

Some cancers are sluggish in spreading to neighboring tissues, while other types move rapidly. Each type of cancer has its own personality so that what is effective therapy against one type may be useless against another.

Between 80 and 90 percent of human cancers are caused by environmental factors, according to Tomotori Mitsuoka, Chief Scientist at the Rikagaku Research Institute in Japan. These carcinogens are generated in the environment or are ingested as precancer-causing substances which become cancer-causing inside the body.[2] Intestinal bacteria play an important part in either the inactivation or the spread of these carcinogens, especially the conversion from nitrosamines, biliary steroids and so on into cancer-causing substances.

Researchers believe that some of the intestinal bacteria are latent pathogenic bacteria, which invade the organs outside the intestinal tract and cause pathological symptoms when the resistance of the host diminishes. Most of the bacteria separated from the focal infection of sepsis, endocarditis, brain tumor, liver tumor, lung tumor, meningitis, urinary tract infection, vaginitis, etc. are those existing as the intestinal resident bacteria. Mitsuoka said it is assumed that some intestinal resident bacteria penetrate the intestinal tract and become a starting point for a disease because of antibiotics, immunity-suppressing substances and cortisone, radiation treatment and physical and psychological stresses.

"Specific and nonspecific irritations of the defense mechanism are not always beneficial to the host. If some of the intestinal bacteria are common to other antigens [allergens] against the infection, they may cause a specific sensitivity that results in asthma, rheumatism, etc.

"Intestinal flora are related to the nutrition, aging, immunity, infections, etc., of the host, suggesting that the intestinal bacteria act as though they are an organ of the body. Therefore, the control of the intestinal bacteria may become either beneficial or harmful to the host. Obviously, the healthier the intestinal bacteria, the healthier and longer lived will be the human host."

COLON CANCER

Lactobacillus acidophilus may prevent cancer of the colon, according to B. R. Goldin and colleagues in the *American Journal of Clinical Nutrition*. Their study involved 21 healthy volunteers who were given *Lactobacillus acidophilus* cultures with milk in concentrations that are similar to those found in acidophilus milk or yogurt to which *Lactobacillus acidophilus* has been added. The researchers reported that after one month, the fecal concentrations of bacterial enzymes that accelerate the conversion of procarcinogens to carcinogens were considerably reduced. This was not true for regular milk without the acidophilus.[3]

Lactobacillic cultures synthesize components which have an antitumor effect, according to scientists at the University of Nebraska in Lincoln. In their study, one group of mice was given plain drinking water, while another group drank water with yogurt in it. Otherwise, the animals ate the same diet. All of the mice were then inoculated with cancer cells. After eight days, 28 percent of the cancer cells in the yogurt-eating mice did not grow, while all of the tumors in the non-yogurt-eating mice continued to proliferate.[4]

In *Infection*, S. L. Gorbach reported that a link between diet and colon cancer is partially due to the alterations in fecal bacterial enzyme activity that results from the Western-type diet. However, in experimental animals at least, these alterations can be normalized by the addition of *Lactobacillus acidophilus* to the diet.[5]

Several types of lactic acid bacteria have been shown to produce anticarcinogenic or antimutagenic activity, according to S. E. Gilliland, Ph.D. in the *Journal of Dairy Science*. These transactions are reportedly due to compounds or substances produced by the organism during growth. He added that there is a possibility that the overall action may be due to antagonistic action of the lactic acid bacteria, especially during growth in the intestines, toward those organisms that might convert procarcinogens into carcinogens.[6]

More evidence that acidophilus is effective against colon cancer has been shown in studies at the Sloan-Kettering Institute of Cancer Research in New York,[7] by G. V. Reddy and colleagues reporting in the *Journal of the National Cancer Institute*, [8] and by British researchers who studied 44 patients with colon cancer and 90 who were disease-free. And evidence supports the fact that populations which consume relatively high quantities of cultured milk products have lower levels of cancer incidence.

A danger of dysbiosis, that is, a disturbance in the ecology of the bowel, is that it produces a large number of highly toxic and sometimes carcinogenic substances in the intestines. Enzyme-producing bacteria convert relatively harmless chemical byproducts of digestion (procarcinogens) into deleterious carcinogens. However, certain enzymes have a lower degree of activity when the bowel receives supplemental acidophilus.

Why are the "friendly" bacteria so successful in fighting some carcinogens?

1. They eliminate substances which can become carcinogenic, such as nitrites. These substances, found in cured meats and other foods, convert into potentially dangerous nitrosamines in the gut. Lactobacilli deactivate nitrates and nitrites before they are converted into nitrosamines.

2. They alter the enzymes produced by other bacteria in the GI tract which convert procarcinogens into carcinogens.

3. They seem to suppress some tumor activity.

BREAST CANCER

Jonathan V. Wright, M.D. says it's no longer a joke to think that "intestinal toxemia" may be related to other diseases, including cancer. In *Dr. Wright's Guide to Healing Nutrition*, he discussed a study at the University of California in San Francisco, in which Nicholas L. Petrakis, Ph.D. studied the cells in breast fluid taken from nonlactating women without cancer. These cells were classified as either normal or showing dysplasia. Dr. Petrakis found that "There was a significant positive association with dysplasia . . . in women reporting severe constipation, i.e., two or fewer bowel movements weekly, which was not seen in women reporting more than one bowel movement daily." Those who had one bowel movement daily or one every other day had less chance of cell dysplasia.[9]

Wright added that men and women who are constipated often have low stomach acidity. Whatever the origin of the constipation, perhaps breast disease should be added to the list of conditions that are believed to be influenced by diet and bowel function, said Wright.

In the Dec. 8, 1969, issue of the *Journal of the American Medical Association*, a Missouri doctor asked about the advisability of applying "dried yogurt" as a therapeutic measure in treating breast cancer. A representative of the American Cancer Society replied that "yogurt and buttermilk may be used interchangeably" and "are in daily use at Calvary Hospital in the Bronx, New York, a facility for the care of patients with advanced cancer."

The regular consumption of unflavored yogurt, especially those brands containing viable *Lactobacillus acidophilus* and other beneficial strains, are bound to be valuable additions to the diet. Lactic acid bacteria, regardless of their type, may prove to be as valuable as penicillin.

THE GREAT CHOLESTEROL DEBATE

The suspected link between serum cholesterol and heart disease is one of the most hotly debated subjects among doctors, biochemists and nutritionists. The fat-like compound gets its name from the substance that was first isolated from gallstones in the late 1900s. The word "cholesterol" is taken from the Greek word for bile, *chole*, and Greek word for solid, *stereos*. Found in all body tissues, cholesterol is essential for certain biochemical processes, especially the production of sex hormones in humans.[1]

While the debate continues, studies show that between 5 and 13 percent of the American population has difficulty metabolizing cholesterol. Although researchers don't yet know how this inherited problem works, it is well known that many natural substances that don't present serious side effects like many cholesterol-lowing drugs are available to treat the condition. The list is long: vitamin C, niacin (B3), oat bran, rice bran, wheat bran, olive oil, pectin. And *Lactobacillus acidophilus*.[2]

A number of researchers have reported the cholesterol-lowering effects of using yogurt and other lactic-culture fermented products. Studies of pigs (whose intestinal and circulatory systems are similar to humans) at Oklahoma State University in Stillwater by Stanley E. Gilliland, Ph.D. and colleagues,[3] of infants fed a formula containing *Lactobacillus acidophilus* (reported in the *American Journal of Clinical Nutrition* in 1975)[4] and of rats fed skim milk fermented with *Lactobacillus acidophilus* all showed significant lowering of cholesterol levels. As Robert L. Sellars pointed out in *Yogurt: Nutritional and Health Properties*, there are a number of hypotheses relating to lactobacilli and their effect on cholesterol.[5]

An interesting study, which was recapped by Ruth Adams and me in *Health Foods*, was conducted by George V. Mann, M.D. of the Vanderbilt University School of Medicine, Nashville, and Anne Spoerry of the African Medical Research Foundation. Based on 24 volunteers from the Masai tribe in Africa who were fed yogurt for three weeks (with only one day of meat-eating), the study showed that their blood cholesterol levels fell dramatically during the three weeks. Even more surprising, the men who had eaten the most yogurt and put on the most weight had the lowest blood cholesterol of all![6] Marvin L. Speck, Ph.D. of North Carolina State University in Raleigh reviewed this study and reported in *Nutrition News* that: "The authors concluded that the fermented milk furnished a factor(s) that impaired the synthesis of cholesterol and thus led to a lowering of serum cholesterol levels."[7]

Should you be concerned about cholesterol? If you have an elevated cholesterol level, there are numerous natural ways of reducing it, such as lactobacilli. On the other hand, cholesterol may not be the main area of concern, especially if you have low vitamin E levels in the blood. Research by K. Fred Gey, M.D. of the Institute of Biochemistry and Molecular Biology in Berne, Switzerland, showed that low blood levels of vitamin E were more predictive of heart disease risk than high cholesterol and blood pressure.[8]

CANDIDA ALBICANS AND THRUSH

A yeast-like fungus that thrives in warm, moist places, *Candida albicans* causes a vaginitis in women that is also known as candidiasis or a yeast infection. This is the same fungus that is sometimes referred to as *Monilia albicans*, with the infection formerly called moniliasis. (It must be noted that numerous bacteria, along with yeast, cause urinary tract infections in adult women.) *Candida* also causes oral thrush and diaper rash in infants, and oral thrush often occurs as a symptom of AIDS (Acquired Immune Deficiency Syndrome). *Candida* can also affect men as well as women, with men reporting symptoms ranging from nervousness, irritability, depression, joint pains, jock itch or repeated fungal infections such as athlete's foot.

Symptoms of a yeast infection in females include vaginal and vulvar itching, soreness and irritation. The vagina may look red instead of pink. There may be a white, curd-like discharge and sexual relations may be uncomfortable. Approximately 15 percent of women, and 30 percent of pregnant women, may have *C. albicans* in their vagina at any time without showing symptoms of vaginitis. Others suffer from it regularly, sometimes coinciding with their menstrual periods.

There are other causes of vaginal itching, including postmenopausal lessening of estrogen and sensitivities to vaginal sprays or deodorants or bubble baths (in young girls), but infections with yeast or bacteria are responsible for 63 percent of cases, according to the FDA Consumer.[1]

If you suffer from frequent vaginitis, several easy lifestyle changes are recommended: (1) not using tampons or having sexual intercourse during treatment, (2) having your partner checked for the infection, (3) wearing cotton underwear and pantyhose with cotton crotches, (4) practicing good feminine hygiene (wash vulva and anal areas daily; after bowel movements, always wipe from front to back away from the vagina), (5) not douching, and (6) making sure anything that enters the vagina—pessaries, diaphragms and other contraceptive devices—is scrupulously clean.

A weakened immune system can also leave someone prone to yeast or other fungal infections. The immune system can be weakened by chronic illness, malnutrition, the use of birth control pills, chemotherapy or radiation therapy, and old age, causing otherwise harmless bacteria to gain a foothold and create problems. In addition, multiple food allergies, particularly to fermented foods, sugar, dried fruits, mushrooms and melons, and chemical sensitivities to such things as molds in the home or workplace and dried leaves may be a sign of candidiasis. Those with diabetes, kidney ailments, cancer and AIDS are especially vulnerable. So-called opportunistic infections are also possible after treatment with broad-spectrum antibiotics, steroid therapy or transplant operations. Candidiasis is a familiar opportunistic infection.[2,3]

HOW ACIDOPHILUS CAN HELP

Research has shown that Lactobacillus acidophilus produces metabolites that inhibit the growth of Candida albicans.[4] The most effective therapy for a yeast infection is a concentrated form of Lactobacillus acidophilus culture, which can be mixed with yogurt and introduced into the vagina as anti-yeast medications, using an applicator.[5] That was corroborated by original research reported in *Clinical Medicine* where bacteria were applied directly to the inflamed, itching tissues with "good to excellent results."[6] Eighty percent of 94 patients with nonspecific vaginitis reported a marked improvement in symptoms after receiving a vaginal lactobacillus preparation, according to a German study.[7]

However, acidophilus "can be an excellent preventative when eaten," according to Marcia Storch, M.D. of the Columbia University College of Physicians and Surgeons in New York. "Many women find that, when they feel the first twinges of itching, taking frequent doses of concentrated acidophilus in capsule or pill form, plus yogurt, will prevent or cure infections." That was also reported by Thomas E. Will, M.D. in *Lancet* (Sept. 1, 1979) when several women with chronic yeast infections caused by colonization of the colon, which then continually reinfected the vagina, successfully treated themselves with preparations containing viable *Lactobacillus acidophilus* cultures.

One cup of yogurt a day reduced the incidence of vaginitis threefold in a study of women with a history of recurring candidal infections, according to Eileen Hilton, M.D. at the Long Island Jewish Medical Center in New York. The results were so dramatic over the 12 months of study that subjects who had started off with the yogurt therapy refused to switch to the no-yogurt regimen for the second six months.[8]

In *The Yeast Connection*, William G. Crook, M.D. said the growth of *Candida albicans* can be reduced with preparations of *Lactobacillus acidophilus, L. bifidus* and/or *Streptococcus faecalis*.[9] An independent study by Terry Willard, Ph.D. of 36 patients with *Candida* symptoms who took a lactic acid bacteria preparation consisting of *Lactobacillus acidophilus, L. bifidus* and *S. faecalis* reported at least 25 percent improvement, while 33 percent had more than 50 percent improvement.[10] Garlic, garlic powder, garlic oil, garlic extract and preparations containing caprylic acid are also beneficial, Dr. Crook noted.

Acidophilus Treatment of AIDS Patients Given the AIDS patient's weakened immune system, it is easy for opportunistic diseases such as *candidasis* and thrush to take over and impede chances for recovery. Ian Brighthope, M.D. of Australia takes an aggressive anti-*Candida* stance in treating patients with AIDS. In addition to a yeast-free diet, he prescribes acidophilus, garlic, Pau d'Arco and a variety of other supplements. In *The AIDS Fighters*, he said: "The lactobacillus itself suppresses the overgrowth of undesirable germs or bacteria, which can produce gases and toxic, soluble substances in the large bowel. When absorbed, these can cause damage to the body's tissues."[11]

An anti-*Candida* diet, designed to starve the yeast infection so it cannot grow, and vitamin C are some of the recommendations of Robert F. Cathcart, III, M.D., who has treated many AIDS patients. The diet eliminates meat and focuses on fresh vegetables and acidophilus.[12] Laurence Badgley, M.D., author of *Healing AIDS Naturally*, notes that acidophilus gives off lactic acid, promoting an environment where other friendly bacteria can prosper.[13]

DEALING WITH CHRONIC YEAST INFECTIONS

What was once considered a yeast infection, in its chronic form, "has been shown to be a neuroimmune disorder that affects the endocrinologic, immunologic and psychologic make-up of afflicted individuals in profound ways," says Keith W. Sehnert, M.D.[14] One quarter of his patients are males, complaining of prostatitis, cystitis, loss of sex drive, chronic fatigue, depression and other symptoms.

He offers a variety of treatment options, including yeast-killing medication such as nystatin powder, which is taken for 16 weeks; a low-sugar, yeast-free diet; *Lactobacillus acidophilus*; and mineral, vitamin and other nutritional supplements, including extra vitamin C, calcium, magnesium, and caprylic acid. Other recommendations include avoiding antibiotics (unless absolutely necessary), oral contraceptives and corticosteroids during treatment, exercise, stress management, changes in lifestyle and work and home environment. Sometimes certain herbal teas, garlic and essential fatty acids are recommended.

Travelers returning from Third World countries often report that it was an exasperating experience because of recurring bouts of traveler's diarrhea, Montezuma's revenge or other appellation for intestinal discomforts, primarily diarrhea. Whereas natives have developed immunity to local parasites, visiting foreigners are sitting ducks. Of course, diarrhea can also strike at home, picked up at a restaurant, a camping site or when swimming in unclean waters. Especially when traveling away from home, it is prudent to carry along some *Lactobacillus acidophilus* capsules to counteract any bacterial infections.

Diarrhea can also be a symptom of food poisoning, an intolerance to certain food, a side effect of a drug (especially certain antibiotics), associated with anxiety or be part of a more complex condition like colitis. Aside from the cramping, pain and enervating effect of this all-too-common illness, the greatest danger is from dehydration, which can be critical for infants and children or those with malnutrition. If you suffer from chronic diarrhea, or diarrhea alternating with constipation, you need to take this condition seriously to uncover the reason behind your symptoms.

In the 1950s, Don J. Weekes, M.D. of the Department of Surgery at Peter Bent Hospital in Boston treated patients suffering from severe diarrhea with tablets containing *L. acidophilus* and *L. bulgaricus*.[1] During an epidemic of diarrhea in Chicago, doctors in the Department of Gastrointestinal Research at the Medical Research Institute of Michael Reese Hospital prescribed *Lactobacillus acidophilus* capsules for some patients. In most cases, there was rapid improvement in less than 24 hours. Four patients had a recurrence when the acidophilus capsules were stopped too early.[2]

A 1989 study of 72 patients ranging in age from 2 to 70 found that *Lactobacillus acidophilus* supplements lowered diarrhea in 84.6 percent of the participants reporting diarrhea. They also found intestinal gas and flatulence decreased with the use of acidophilus. Studies of childhood diarrhea in 1963 and again in 1987 showed that yogurt provided successful treatment.[3]

Dysentery is a severe form of diarrhea caused by *Salmonella* or *Shigella* organisms. In a study of Polish children afflicted with dysentery, 40 to 70 percent of the children recovered after being fed acidophilus milk compared to the control group.

Andrew Weil, M.D., author of *Natural Health, Natural Medicine*, said that acidophilus supplements provide a much higher concentration of the desired organisms than do yogurt, acidophilus milk and other cultured milk products. It doesn't matter whether the supplements are derived from milk or vegetarian sources, he added; however, check the expiration dates on any acidophilus product to insure the beneficial bacteria are alive.[4]

REPLACING INTESTINAL FLORA AFTER ANTIBIOTIC TREATMENT

The era of modern-day antibiotics began in 1928 when Dr. Alexander Fleming, a British scientist, accidentally discovered penicillin. Since then, thousands of antibiotics have been discovered, though relatively few are in use, and countless lives have been saved.

The problem is when dangerous bacteria become resistant to antibiotics (a phenomenon seen more often today and caused in part by our overuse of antibiotics) and also in their side effects. Antibiotics can cause: diarrhea, constipation, nausea, photosensitive skin reactions, rashes, yeast infections, weight gain, teeth discoloration and depletion of nutrients including vitamins. Also, helpful bacteria in the intestinal tract can be destroyed along with the harmful ones.

However, because antibiotics kill bacteria in the intestine but are not as effective in containing E. coli and Candida albicans, many patients who require antibiotics are at risk of being "overcolonized" by Candida and other undesirable organisms. The remedy? Lactobacillus acidophilus.[1]

"Acidophilus may be used to colonize the intestine with the normal flora," said Abram Hoffer, M.D., Ph.D. "One can use foods rich in these organisms, such as sour milk, naturally fermented yogurt or sauerkraut, or the lactobacillus variants available. . . . They should be taken with each meal and continued for a week after the antibiotic has been stopped."[2]

In Japan, lactic acid bacteria have been used to counteract the side effects of antibiotics prescribed to new mothers to treat urinary tract infections, breast inflammation and other illnesses cause by bacteria. Another Japanese study proved the effectiveness of lactic acid bacteria products against an antibiotic given to children who had a variety of infectious diseases. They had fewer side effects and showed faster improvement. Indeed, researchers at the Department of Food Science and Nutrition at the Ohio Agricultural Research and Development Center in Columbus reported a substance isolated from skim milk cultured with Lactobacillus acidophilus is a potent antibiotic against certain pathogens, including viruses.

If you must take antibiotics, it seems prudent to take Lactobacillus acidophilus and other lactic acid bacteria products before, during and after antibiotic use. These friendly bacteria restore the intestinal flora to pre-antibiotic condition and can help minimize any complications or side effects of the drug.

Two conditions that have been shown to improve upon treatment with acidophilus are lactose intolerance and acne rosacea.

An estimated 30 million Americans have some degree of lactose intolerance, because they do not have the digestive enzyme, lactase, which is necessary to digest lactose (milk sugar). Lactose intolerance is found among 79 percent of Native Americans, 75 percent of African-Americans, 51 percent of Hispanics and 21 percent of Caucasians, according to the United Dairy Industry Association. In some people, lactase production lessens with age. Symptoms include bloating, diarrhea, stomach cramps and other intestinal discomfort after ingesting dairy products.

Intestinal disorders (inflammatory bowel disease), medications (antibiotics and anti-inflammatories) and surgery can also reduce lactase production by the body. Sometimes the lactase deficiency is only temporary. But most people are able to continue to enjoy yogurt. "Some fermented products like yogurt actually digest lactose through the active cultures they contain, so these are more easily handled," said Dennis A. Savaiano, Ph.D. of the Department of Food Science and Nutrition at the University of Minnesota. However, Marvin L. Speck, Ph.D. of North Carolina State University has noted that those who can't digest yogurt can be helped by using acidophilus supplements.[1]

Unfortunately, many people who avoid milk products due to an intolerance are missing the many nutrients available primarily through dairy products. If you want to continue drinking milk, there are several products from the Lactaid company, including lactase you can add as a powder or take in tablet form, or milk already containing lactase. Adding acidophilus to any dairy product will provide an extra boost from this beneficial bacteria.

Acne rosacea (pronounced acne ro-za'-she-ah) is an unsightly skin condition sometimes called "adult acne" to distinguish it from acne vulgaris, or teenage acne. It's characterized by an increase in size and visibility of blood vessels under the skin of the nose, cheeks and forehead, often producing a red blotchy appearance. In men more so than women, the tip of the nose becomes enlarged and bright red, á la the late W. C. Fields, who may have had an advanced case of rosacea.

Since a sluggish digestive system which causes a build-up of toxins is suspected of being behind many common ailments, including skin disorders, *Lactobacillus acidophilus* may be helpful, according to Jonathan V. Wright, M.D. Also, since acne and other skin conditions are often treated with antibiotics, which destroy beneficial bacteria as well as dangerous ones, it's logical that restoring the intestinal flora with acidophilus can help the body's own detoxification processes where they start.[2]

Because antibiotics and topical corticosteroids often prescribed for acne rosacea only serve as a Band-Aid, holistic physicians are more likely to consider remedies such as acidophilus, nutrients including the B vitamins and possibly hydrochloric acid supplements for cases of low stomach acidity that interferes with absorption of nutrients. As with many skin ailments, stress and other lifestyle factors can play an important role in adult acne. To avoid aggravating acne rosacea, you should avoid sun and wind exposure, extreme temperatures, alcohol and spicy foods and extremely hot liquids.

REFERENCES

Introduction
1. Speck, Marvin L., Ph.D. "Contributions of Microorganisms to Foods and Nutrition," *Nutrition News*, vol. 38, no. 4 (December 1975).
2. Brochu, Edouard. "Special Behavior of Lactic Bacteria and Their Relation to Nutrition and Health." Paper read at the Canadian Health Food Association convention, Aug. 10, 1986.
3. Mitsuoka, Tomotori, M.D. "Intestinal Bacteria Flora and Its Significance," *Clinics and Bacteria*, vol. 2, no. 3, Sept. 20, 1975.

The Benefits of Yogurt
1. Hauser, Gayelord. *Look Younger, Live Longer*. New York: Farrar, Straus, 1950.
2. Hirshberg, Meg Cadoux. *The Stonyfield Farm Yogurt Cookbook*. Charlotte, Vt.: Camden House Publishing, 1991.
3. Burke, Peter F. "How Yogurt Is Made," undated.
4. Hendler, Sheldon Saul, M.D., Ph.D. *The Purification Prescription*. New York: William Morrow, 1991.
5. Chandan, Ramesh C., Ph.D., ed. *Yogurt: Nutritional and Health Properties*. McLean, Va.: National Yogurt Association, 1989.
6. Chaitow, Leon, N.D., D.O., and Trenev, Natasha. *ProBiotics*. Wellingborough, England: Thorsons Publishing Group, 1990.
7. Hausman, Patricia, and Hurley, Judith Benn. *The Healing Foods*. Emmaus, Penn.: Rodale Press, 1989.
8. Reuben, Carolyn, C.A., and Priestley, Joan, M.D. *Essential Supplements for Women*. New York: Putnam's/Perigee, 1988.

Two Men Behind the Microbes
1. Slosson, Edwin E., M.S., Ph.D. *Major Prophets of To-Day*. Boston: Little, Brown, 1914.

Improving Digestion
1. Ensminger, Audrey H., et al. *Foods and Nutrition Encyclopedia*. Clovis, Calif.: Pegus Press, 1983.
2. Hoffer, Abram, M.D., Ph.D, *Orthomolecular Medicine for Physicians*. New Canaan, Conn.: Keats Publishing, 1989.
3. Barnard, Christiaan, M.D., and Illman, John. *The Body Machine*. New York: Crown Publishers, 1981.

ACIDOPHILUS AND YOUR HEALTH / 43

4. Yudkin, John, M.D. *The Penguin Encyclopedia of Nutrition*. New York: Viking Press, 1985.
5. Werbach, Melvyn R., M.D. *Nutritional Influences on Illness*. New Canaan, Conn.: Keats Publishing, 1989.
6. Rettger, L. F., et al. *Lactobacillus acidophilus: Its Therapeutic Application*. New Haven, Conn.: Yale University Press, 1935.
7. *Lancet General Advertiser*, Sept. 21, 1957.
8. Weinstein, L., M.D., et al. "Therapeutic Application of Acidophilus Milk in Simple Constipation," *Arch. Intern. Med.* 52: 384 (1933).
9. Kopeloff, N. "Clinical Results Obtained with Bacillus Acidophilus," *Arch. Intern. Med.* 33: 47 (1924).
10. *Lancet General Advertiser, op. cit.*
11. Niv, M. et al. "Yogurt in the Treatment of Infantile Diarrhea," *Clin. Ped.* 2: 407-11 (1963).
12. Winkelstein, Asher, M.D. "*Lactobacillus acidophilus* Tablets in the Therapy of Functional Disorders," *Amer. Pract. & Digest of Treat.*, October 1956, pp. 1637-39.
13. Crook, William G., M.D. *The Yeast Connection: A Medical Breakthrough*. Jackson, Tenn.: Professional Books, 1984.
14. Roth, James L. A., M.D., and Levitt, Michael D., M.D. *Medical World News*, April 21, 1975.
15. "Special Report on Acidophilus Milk: Sorting Out the Truth Behind the Health Claims," *Diveronm. Nutrition*, April 1987.
16. Smith, Lendon, M.D. *Feed Yourself Right*. New York: Dell Publishing, 1983.
17. Murray, Frank. "Acidophilus May Improve Your Digestion," *Better Nutrition*, December 1984.
18. Honma, N. et al. "Clinical Effects of Lactic Acid Bacteria," *New Medicines & Clinics*, vol. 36, no. 1 (Jan. 10, 1987).
19. Bricklin, Mark. *The Practical Encyclopedia of Natural Healing*. New York: Penguin Books, 1990.

Cancer and the Effects of Acidophilus

1. Lewis, Howard R., and Lewis, Martha E. *The People's Medical Manua*. Garden City, N.Y.: Doubleday, 1986.
2. Mitsuoka, Tomotori. "Intestinal Bacteria Flora and Its Significance," *Clinics and Bacteria*, vol., 2, no. 3, Sept. 20, 1975.
3. Goldin, B. R., and Gorbach, S. L. "The Effect of Milk and Lactobacillus Feeding on Human Intestinal Bacterial Enzyme Activity," *Amer. J. Clin. Nutr.* 39 (1984): 756-61.
4. Adams, Ruth and Murray, Frank. *Health Foods*. New York: Larchmont Books, 1983.
5. Gorbach, S. L. "The Intestinal Microflora and Its Colon Cancer Connection," *Infection* 10(6): 379-84 (1982).
6. Gilliland, S. E. "Acidophilus Milk Products: A Review of Potential Benefits to Consumers," *J. Dairy Sci.* 72: 2483-94 (1989).
7. Lee, William H., R.Ph.D., *The Friendly Bacteria*. New Canaan, Conn.: Keats Publishing, 1988.
8. Reddy, G. V., et al. "Inhibitory Effect of Yogurt on Ehrlich Ascites Tumor-Cell Proliferation," *J. Nat. Cancer Inst.* 50: 815-17 (1973).

9. Wright, Jonathan V., M.D. *Dr. Wright's Guide to Healing with Nutrition.* New Canaan, Conn.: Keats Publishing, 1990.

The Great Cholesterol Debate
1. Ensminger, Audrey H., et al. *Foods and Nutrition Encyclopedia.* Clovis, Calif.: Pegus Press, 1983.
2. Murray, Frank. *Program Your Heart for Health.* New York: Larchmont Books, 1978.
3. Altschule, Mark D., M.D. "How Little We Know" in *Medical and Health Annual.* Chicago: Encyclopedia Britannica, 1980.
4. Gilliland, S. E. "Acidophilus Milk Products: A Review of Potential Benefits to Consumers," *J. Dairy Sci.* 72: 2483-94 (1989).
5. Sellars, Robert L. "Health Properties of Yogurt" in *Yogurt: Nutritional and Health Properties,* Ramesh C. Chandan, Ph.D., ed. McLean, Va.: National Yogurt Association, 1989.
6. Adams, Ruth and Murray, Frank. *Health Foods.* New York: Larchmont Books, 1983.
7. Speck, Marvin L., Ph.D. "Contributions of Microorganisms to Foods and Nutrition," *Nutrition News,* December 1975.
8. "Vitamin E Studied in Cardiac Death," *Med. Trib.,* Feb. 7, 1991.

Candida Albicans and Thrush
1. Zamula, Evelyn. "On Yeast Infections and Other Female Irritations," *FDA Consumer,* July-August 1985.
2. Subak-Sharpe, Genell J., et al. *The Physicians' Manual for Patients.* New York: New York Times Books, 1984.
3. Wunderlich, Ray C., Jr., and Kalita, Dwight K., Ph.D. *Candida Albicans.* New Canaan, Conn.: Keats Publishing, 1984.
4. Collins, E. B., and Hardt, Pamela. "Inhibition of Candida Albicans by *Lactobacillus acidophilus,*" *J. Dairy Sci.* 63: 830-32 (1980).
5. Bricklin, Mark, et al. *Encyclopedia of Natural Healing.* Emmaus, Penna.: Rodale Press, 1983.
6. Adam, Ruth and Murray, Frank. *Health Foods.* New York: Larchmont Books, 1983.
7. Fernandes, C. F., et al. "Therapeutic Role of Dietary Lactobacilli and Lactobacillic Fermented Dairy Products," *FEMS Microbiol. Revs.* (Federation of European Microbiological Societies) 46: 343-56 (1987).
8. Crook, William G., M.D. *The Yeast Connection.* Jackson, Tenn.: Professional Books, 1986.
9. Karkut, G. "Effect of Lactobacillus Immunotherapy on Genital Infections in Women," *Geburtshilfe Fraunheilkd* 44(5): 311-14 (1984).
10. Barkhead, Charles D. "Yogurt Wins Points in Test Against Recurring Vaginitis," *Med. World News,* Oct. 23, 1989.
11. Willard, Terry, Ph.D. "Kyo-Dophilus Use in the Reduction of *Candida albicans* Symptoms," unpublished paper, Jan. 28, 1989.
12. Brighthope, Ian, M.D. and Fitzgerald, Peter. *The AIDS Fighters.* New Canaan, Conn.: Keats Publishing, 1987.

13. Badgley, Laurence, M.D. *Healing AIDS Naturally.* San Bruno, Calif.: Human Energy Press, 1986.
14. Murray, Frank. "Vitamin C: A Clue for AIDS Treatment," *Better Nutrition,* Sept. 1987.

Diarrhea
1. Bricklin, Mark, et al. *The Practical Encyclopedia of Natural Healing.* Emmaus, Penna.: Rodale Press, 1983.
2. Beck, Charles, M.D., and Necheles, H., M.D., Ph.D. "Beneficial Effects of Administration of *Lactobacillus acidophilus* in Diarrheal and Other Intestinal Disorders," *Amer. J. Gastroenter.* 35: 522-30 (1961).
3. Antoine, Jean M. "Validation of Health Attributes of Yogurt" in *Yogurt: Nutritional and Health Properties.* Ramesh C. Chandan, Ph.D., ed. McLean, Va.: National Yogurt Association, 1989.
4. Weil, Andrew, M.D. *Natural Health, Natural Medicine.* Boston: Houghton Mifflin, 1990.

Replacing Intestinal Flora After Antibiotic Treatment
1. Atkins, Robert C., M.D. *Dr. Atkins' Nutrition Breakthrough.* New York: William Morrow, 1981.
2. Hoffer, Abram, M.D., Ph.D. *Orthomolecular Medicine for Physicians.* New Canaan, Conn.: Keats Publishing, 1989.
3. Katagiri, Seiichi, M.D. "Study on Anti-Diarrhea Effect: Combined Use of Augmentin and Lactic Acid Bacteria Product of Multiple Resistance," *Basics and Clinics* 20(7): 651-53 (Dec. 1986).
4. Kanki, Kozo, M.D., et al. "Effects of Cepoperazone on the Intestinal Bacteria Flora and Occurrence of Diarrhea in Children," *J. Infect. Dis.* Nov. 20, 1987, pp. 1257-62.
5. Hamdan, I. Y., and Mikolajcik, E. M. "Acidolin: An Antibiotic Produced by *Lactobacillus acidophilus,*" *J. Antibiotics* 27(8): 631-36 (1974).

Other Conditions Helped by Acidophilus
1. Adams, Ruth and Murray, Frank. *Health Foods.* New York: Larchmont Books, 1983.
2. Wright, Jonathan V., M.D. *Dr. Wright's Guide to Healing with Nutrition.* New Canaan, Conn.: Keats Publishing, 1990.